Natural Hair Care Recipes

A Complete Collection of DIY, Homemade Ideas!

Table of Contents

Conditioners are an important part of hair care, too. They help your hair to deal with the stresses it faces every day. Here are some of the best DIY choices… 53

Introduction

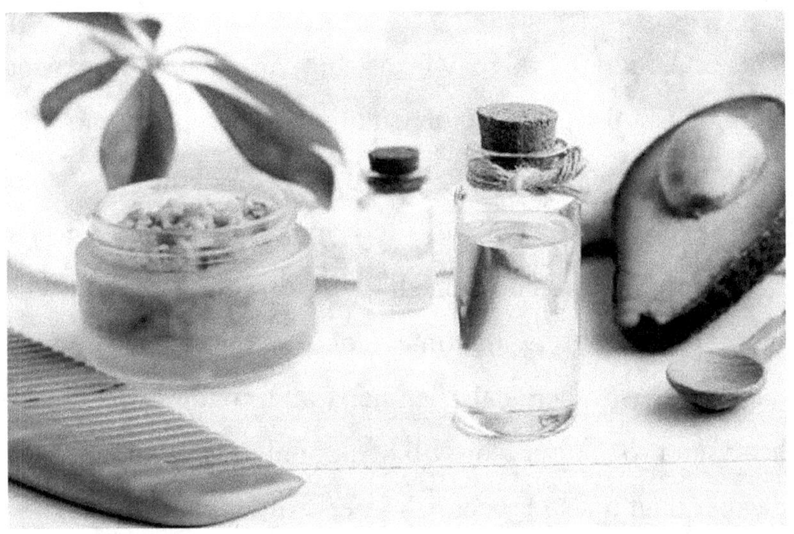

Do you want to make the switch from commercial hair products to those made at home using natural ingredients?

Homemade shampoos and conditioners can rejuvenate your silky hair without stripping its natural oils or adding chemicals to the equation.

Please note, right up front, that if you have been using conventional hair products for years, it will take time for it to adjust to natural products you make at home. This transition period is a detox phase where your scalp and hair become accustomed to the natural ingredients. It will produce more sebum for a time.

This transition period may be as short as a couple weeks, or as long as a few months, depending on the type of hair you have, its texture and the new ingredients you are using. You'll need to be patient, to allow your hair the time it needs to become accustomed to healthy ingredients. Your hair will likely be oily during this time. Don't let that make you turn back to harsh chemical shampoos and conditioners. Take heart, and soon your hair will be not only beautiful, but also cleaner than it's ever been, and free from toxins.

Making your own shampoo and conditioner is an excellent way to provide your hair with the nutrients it needs, without including the chemicals it doesn't. The homemade recipes in this book will utilize many ingredients you already have at home. So they're easy to make and they save money, too. Give your hair a natural clean with homemade shampoos and conditioners.

The first step in most hair care regimens is shampoo. Here are some recipes for shampoos that will help keep your hair healthy...

1 – Homemade Castile Shampoo for Normal Hair

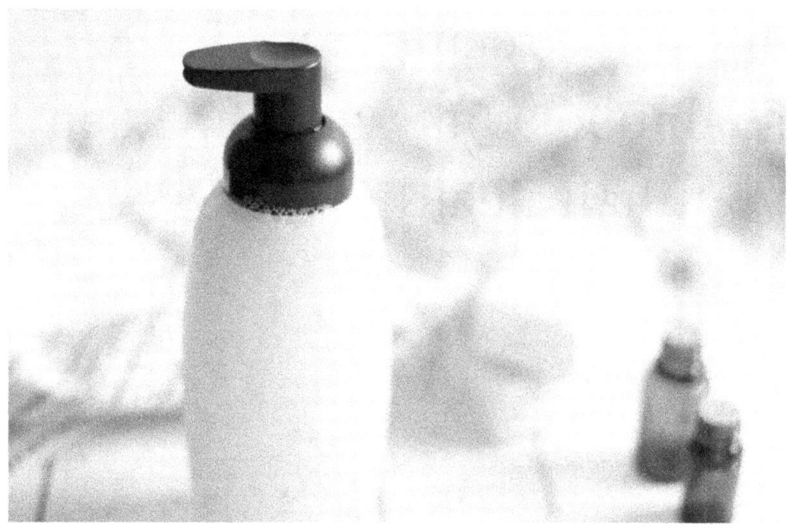

This natural shampoo works wonderfully on normal hair. You can also use it as a starter recipe, and add your favorite scent. You'll get some rich lather from this shampoo, even though it's still less than you get from commercial shampoos – chemicals give more lather, but it comes at a price.

Makes 1/2 cup

Prep Time: 5 minutes

Ingredients:

- 1/4 cup of water, distilled
- 1/4 cup of castile soap, liquid, unscented
- 1/2 tsp. of grapeseed or jojoba oil (carrier oil)

Instructions:

1. Mix all ingredients and pour into a plastic bottle.

2. Shake before each use. This shampoo is not as thick as you're accustomed to with commercial products. Just tilt your bottle to get it to pour on your hair.

2 – DIY Shampoo for Proper PH Balance

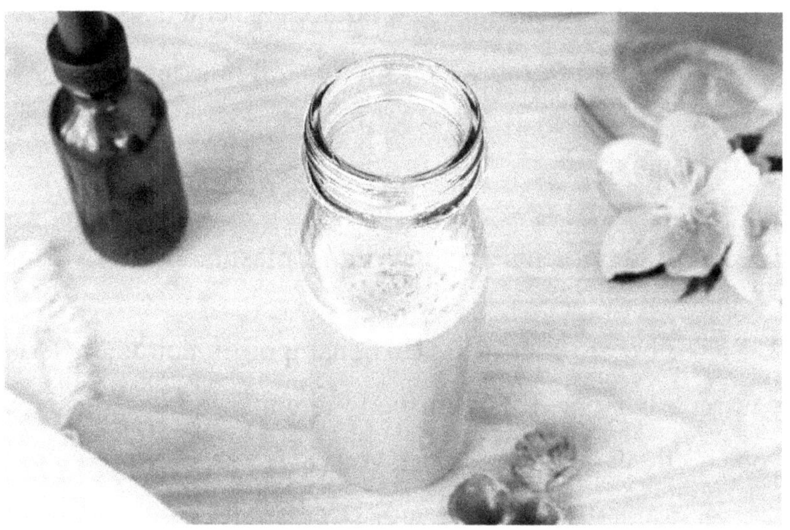

This DIY shampoo is PH balanced, and you should be able to keep the bottle in the shower. I always put it in my refrigerator, though, so it will last longer. Alternately, you can make a larger batch by pouring the mixture in ice cube trays. Then you can freeze it until you need it, and the batch will last longer.

Makes about 15 ounces

Prep Time: 10-15 minutes

Ingredients:

- 1 x 14-oz. can of coconut milk, full fat
- 2 tbsp. of honey, raw, liquid
- 1 tsp. of oil, jojoba (carrier oil)
- 1 tsp. of castor oil
- 2 tbsp. of vinegar, apple cider
- 1 tsp. of essential oil, your choice – tea tree, cedarwood and lavender work well

Instructions:

1. Combine the ingredients in medium bowl. Whisk mixture till you have a smooth texture. It will separate a bit, so you'll need to shake it well before you use it.

2. For use, massage small amount of shampoo on your scalp. Use a comb or your fingers to work it into your hair. Leave it sit for several minutes before you rinse it off.

3. If you have naturally oily hair, you can follow this shampoo with a rinse made with water and apple cider vinegar.

3 – Homemade Stimulation Shampoo

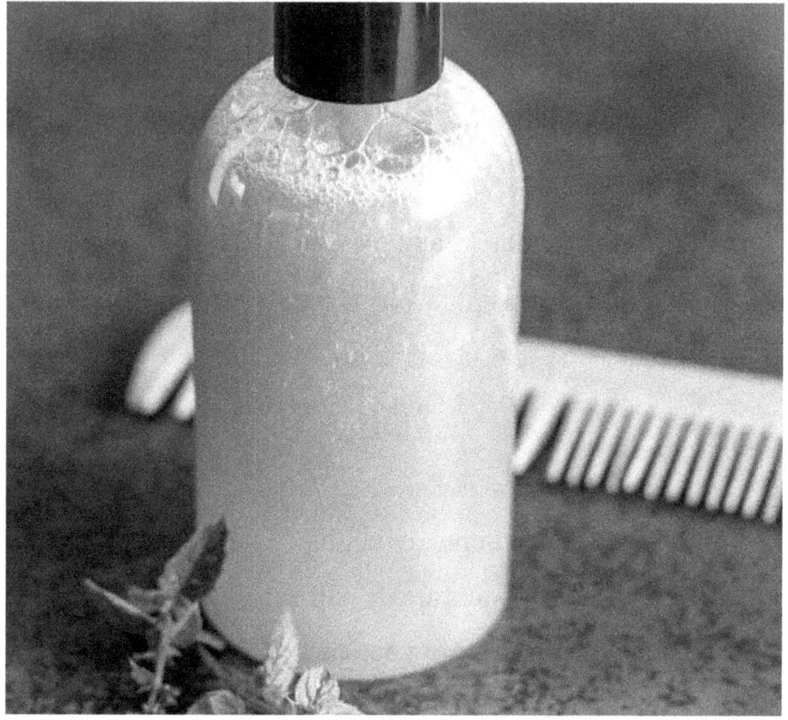

This shampoo will wake up your senses, as well as your scalp. The peppermint and tea tree oil work together to make that possible. This is a gentle shampoo, so you can use it every day. You'll enjoy the refreshing nature of the blend.

Makes 1/2 cup

Prep Time: 10 minutes

Ingredients:

- 1/4 cup castile soap, liquid
- 1/4 cup of water, distilled
- 1/2 tsp. of oil, neutral carrier, like jojoba, etc.
- 1/8 tsp. of tea tree oil
- 1/8 tsp. of peppermint oil

Instructions:

1. Mix the ingredients well and store mixture in plastic bottle. Use just like you would use any other shampoo and rinse your hair well.

4 – DIY Peppermint & Rosemary Shampoo

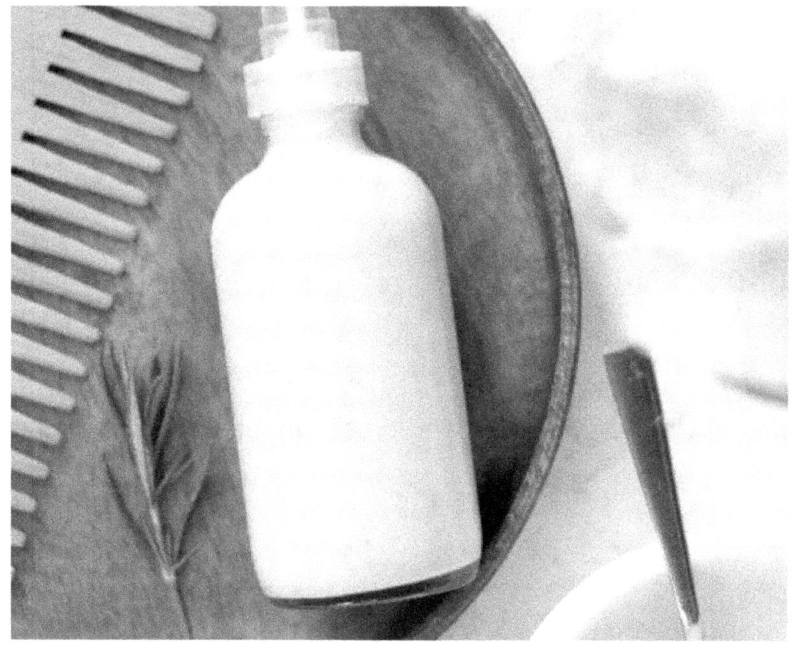

When you use essential oils in your DIY shampoos, you'll fine that they work excellently for cleansing, strengthening and nourishing your scalp and hair. Peppermint and rosemary essential oils not only help to get rid of excess oil in the hair – they also boost your alertness and mental clarity.

Makes about 1 cup

Prep Time: 5 minutes

Ingredients:

- 1/2 cup of water, filtered or distilled
- 1/2 cup of soap, Castile
- 2 drops of peppermint oil
- 16 drops of rosemary oil

Instructions:

1. Add castile soap to flip top container.

2. Add peppermint and rosemary essential oils.

3. Add filtered water.

4. To use this shampoo, apply several squirts to your hair. Shampoo and then rinse as you normally would.

5 – Homemade Moisturizing Shampoo

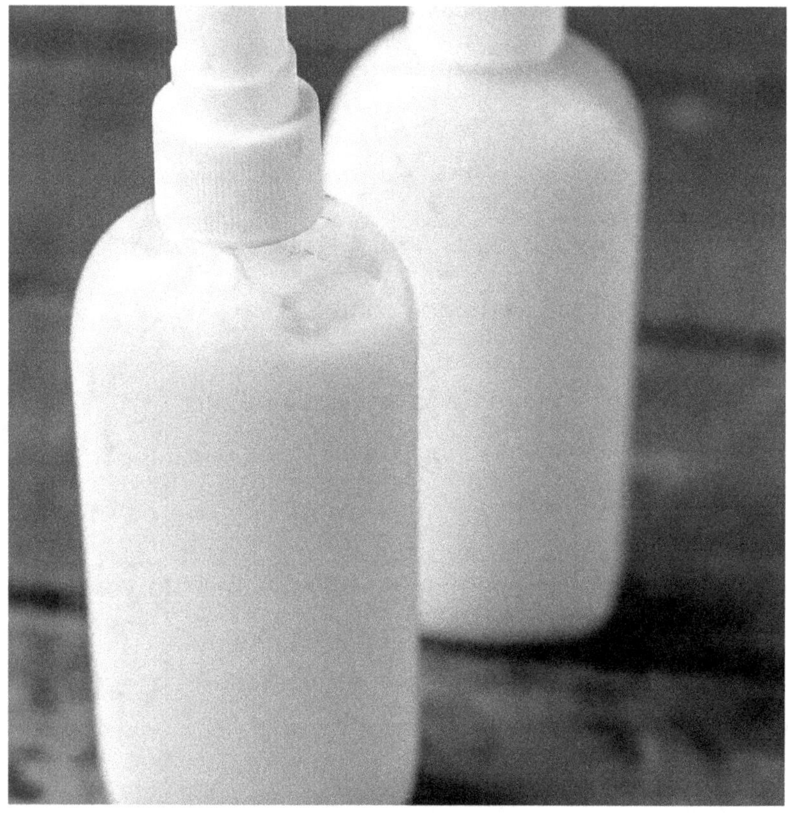

This shampoo will not offer you the same lather as commercial products, but it cleanses and moisturizes naturally. Don't use a lot, or it may leave residue behind in your hair. You can replace commercial shampoos with homemade versions like this gradually, so your hair can adjust, making the transition easier.

Makes 3/4 cup

Prep Time: 10 minutes

Ingredients:

- 1/4 cup of water, distilled
- 1/4 cup of Aloe Vera gel
- 1/4 cup of castile soap, liquid, in your fav. scent
- 1 tsp. of glycerin
- 1/4 tsp. of jojoba or avocado oil

Instructions:

1. Mix all the ingredients together. Store the shampoo in a plastic squeeze bottle, if you have one, and shake it well before you use it.

2. Apply shampoo to hair and leave it sit for several minutes, then rinse it out well using cool (not warm) water.

6 – DIY Maple Syrup Shampoo

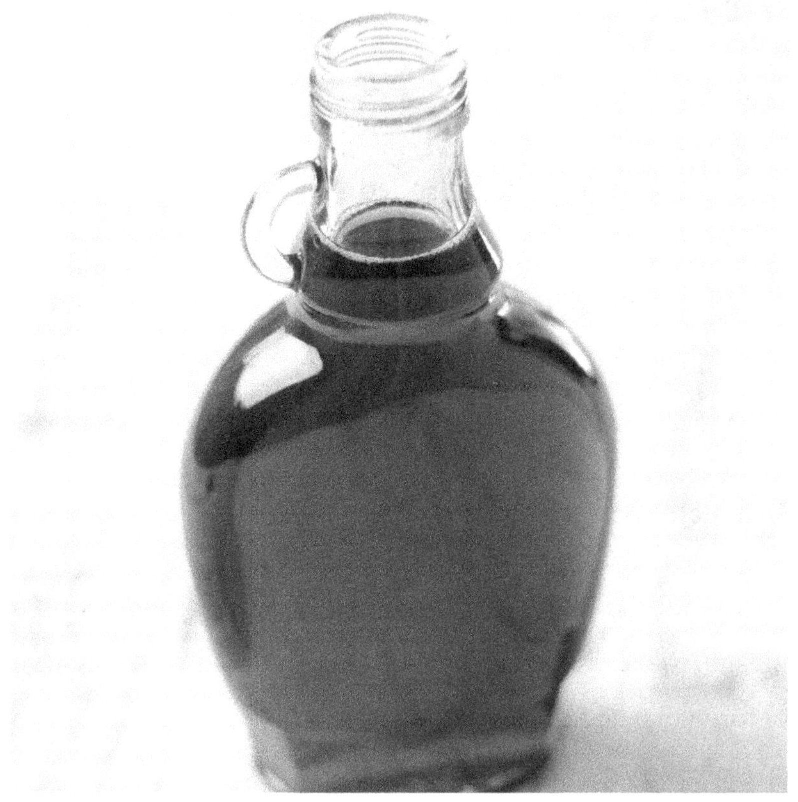

Enhancing the natural growth of your hair is the reason this recipe was created. The ingredients are affordable and easy to find. This shampoo smells terrific and helps hair to grow thicker and faster. It's mild, too, so you can use it every day.

Makes about 1/2 cup

Prep Time: 5 minutes

Ingredients:

- 2 tbsp. of syrup, maple
- 1/2 cup of Castile soap, liquid
- 10 drops castor oil
- 10 drops carrot seed essential oil

Instructions:

1. Mix the ingredients well. Store in heavy plastic bottle to increase the shampoo shelf life.

7 – Soothing Homemade Shampoo

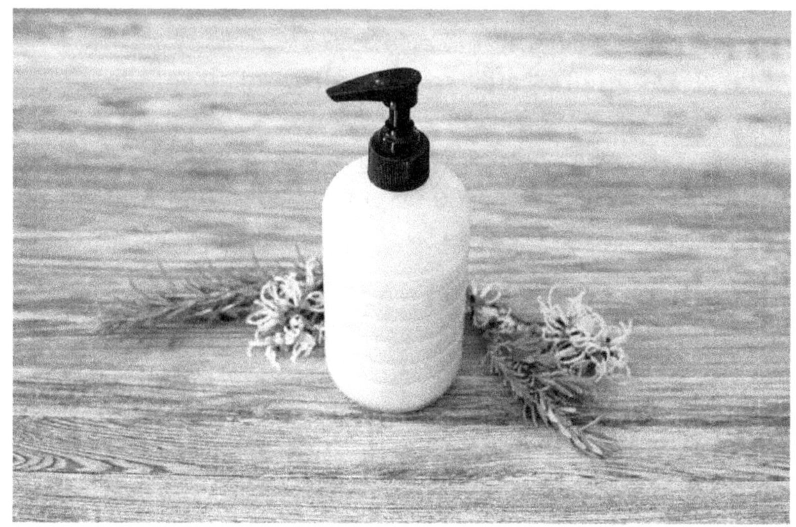

This recipe uses chamomile to calm your hair and scalp. It has lightening properties that come natural to this essential oil, so add lemon juice to the mix if you'd like to lighten your hair a bit.

Makes 2 cups

Prep Time: 10 minutes

Ingredients:

- 1 cup of castile, soap, lavender
- 1 cup of water, distilled

- 1 & 1/2 tbsp. of glycerin

- 6 tea bags, chamomile

Instructions:

1. Steep tea bags in a cup of boiled water for 15-20 minutes. Remove tea bags, then discard them.

2. Add the castile soap to tea. Add glycerin till blended well. Store in cool, dark place in well-sealed bottle.

8 – DIY Green Tea Shampoo

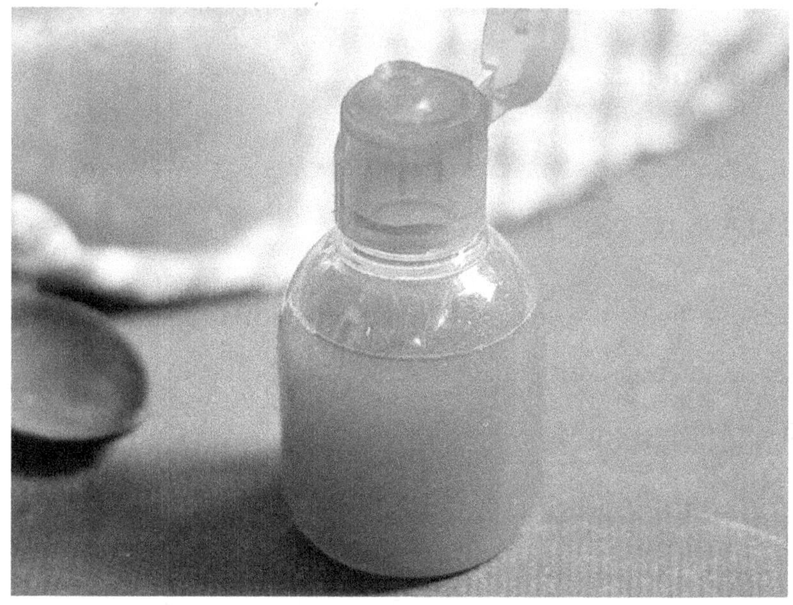

The more you know about the chemicals in commercial shampoo, the more you may want to question those products, and change the way you live your life. You can make natural choices in the products you use. Making your own shampoo is just one way to make the change to natural products in your life.

Makes about 2 cups

Prep Time: 5 minutes + 30 minutes brewing time

Ingredients:

- 1 cup of tea, green – allow to brew for 1/2 hour before using
- 1 cup of pure castile soap liquid
- 1 tbsp. of olive oil, organic
- 1 tsp. of honey, raw, organic

Instructions:

1. Brew the tea for 1/2 hour.

2. Add in the rest of the ingredients.

3. Mix well and then add the essential oils.

9 – Homemade Dandruff Repair Shampoo

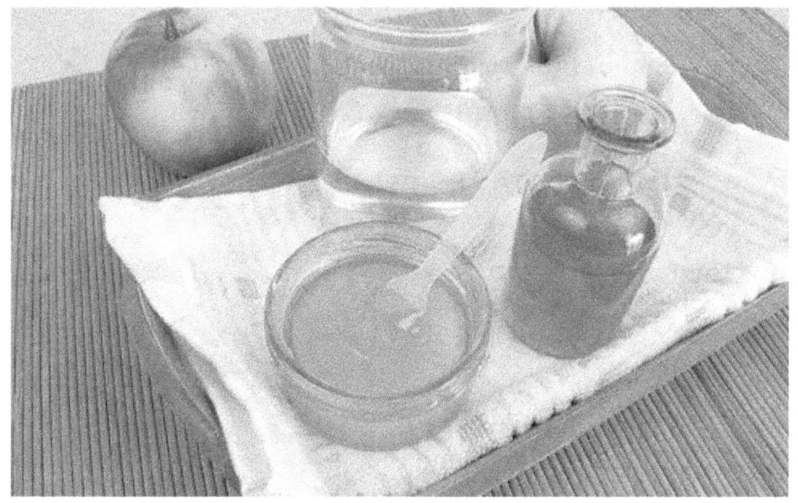

Anyone, at any age, can have dandruff. It may cause a dry, flaky scalp or an oily, flaky scalp. Improperly caring for hair won't cause dandruff. Using a natural shampoo will help ease the stress that affects your hair every day, and clear up dandruff without toxic chemicals.

Makes 3/4 cup

Prep Time: 10 minutes

Ingredients:

- 1/4 cup of castile soap, liquid
- 1/4 cup of water, distilled
- 1 tbsp. of vinegar, apple cider
- 1/2 tsp. of grapeseed or jojoba oil
- 6 cloves, ground finely
- 3 tbsp. of apple juice, pure

Instructions:

1. In small sized blender or grinder, mix all the ingredients on a low setting for 1/2 minute.

2. Wet your hair using warm water. Massage shampoo into your hair well, then rinse it out using warm water. Cover leftover shampoo and keep it in the fridge. Throw out after three days' storage.

10 – Honey & Carrot Seed Oil DIY Shampoo

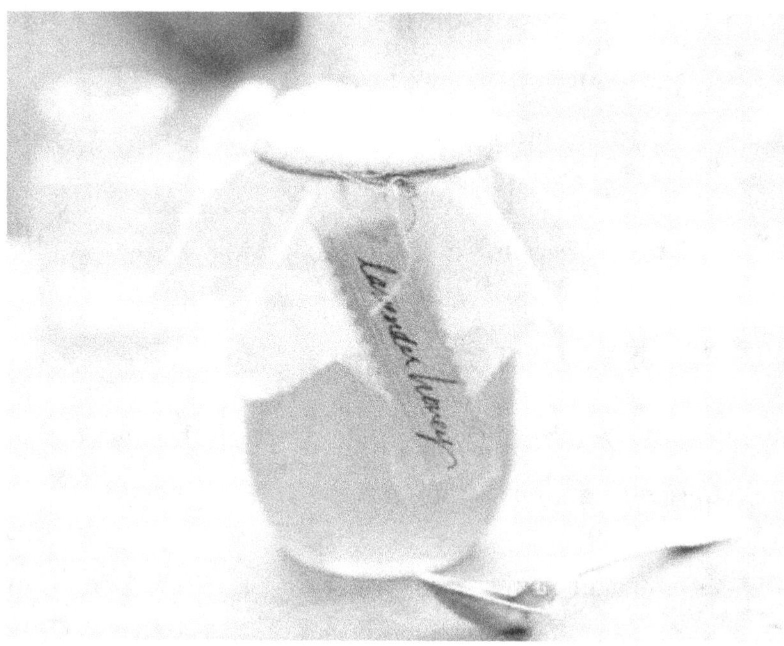

This honey-based shampoo is a luxurious way to give you shiny, soft hair that can even become more wavy or curly than it is naturally. It also helps in getting rid of frizzies. It aids the oil production of your scalp in normalizing, and you'll be able to go for more days between washing your hair.

Makes about 3 tbsp.

Prep Time: 15 minutes

Ingredients:

- 3 tbsp. of water, filtered
- 1 tbsp. of honey, raw
- Several drops of carrot seed oil + any other essential oils you like

Instructions:

1. Use the amounts above to make one serving of this shampoo at a time, so extra won't spoil.

2. Add essential oils to the shampoo, your favorite types. These oils help with flaky scalp problems and add a pleasing fragrance. Carrot seed oil is quite nourishing for your hair.

3. If you need to, the mixture can be heated on low heat so the honey dissolves better.

4. The shampoo will be quite watery – that's normal.

5. Wet your hair. Massage a small amount of shampoo on your scalp. Massage and distribute well. Rinse well.

11 – Homemade Cocoa Dry Shampoo

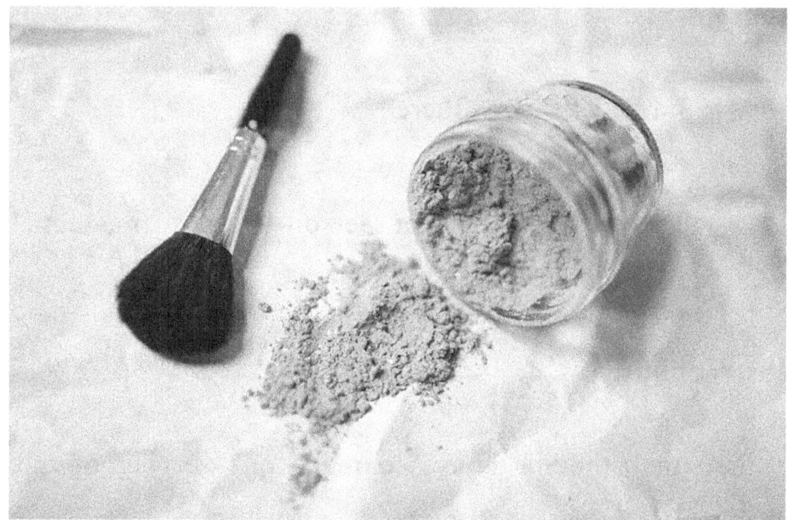

Making dry shampoo that is natural and organic is easy to do. You can make up a batch in just part of one afternoon. The process is easily followed and will yield balanced, healthier, stronger hair. Plus, it will retain these positive properties without using harmful chemicals. This also helps your hair to retain its natural color and body.

Makes about 1/2 cup

Prep Time: 10 minutes

Ingredients:

- 2 tbsp. cocoa powder, organic
- 1/4 cup corn starch
- 5-8 drops lavender essential oil
- 5 drops almond, orange, lemon, rose, bergamot, eucalyptus or tea tree essential oils

Instructions:

1. Mix dry ingredients together in bowl with spoon or whisk.

2. Add essential oils as you stir, and cover remainder of mixture.

12 – DIY Calendula & Sage Herbal Shampoo

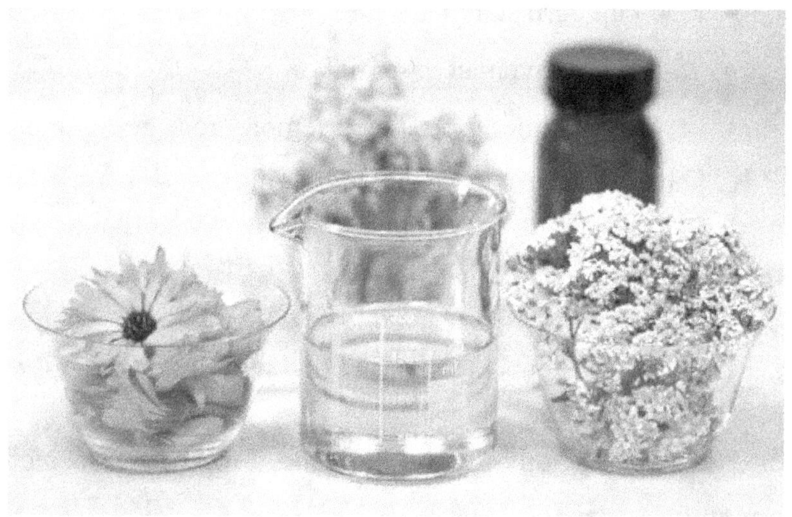

When you make your shampoo at home, you'll find it isn't as easy to work up a lather as it is with commercial products. But it still cleans hair – it just uses botanicals and nourishing ingredients, instead of chemicals, so it's gentler on your hair. Your hair won't be as squeaky clean as you are accustomed to, but that's because natural shampoos won't strip your hair's natural oils.

Makes about 10 ounces

Prep Time: 10-12 minutes + 4 hours steeping time

Ingredients:

- 8 ounces of water, filtered
- 3 ounces of castile soap, liquid
- 1 to 2 tbsp. of sage and organic calendula herbs, dried
- 1/4 tsp. of olive or jojoba oil – if your hair is normally dry, use more

Instructions:

1. Make herbal infusion. Pour boiling hot water over herbs and cover. Let them steep for four hours or more.

2. Strain out herbs. Pour reserved liquid in plastic bottle. Add oils and castile soap.

3. Shake well before using, since these contents separate naturally.

13 – Homemade Beer Shampoo

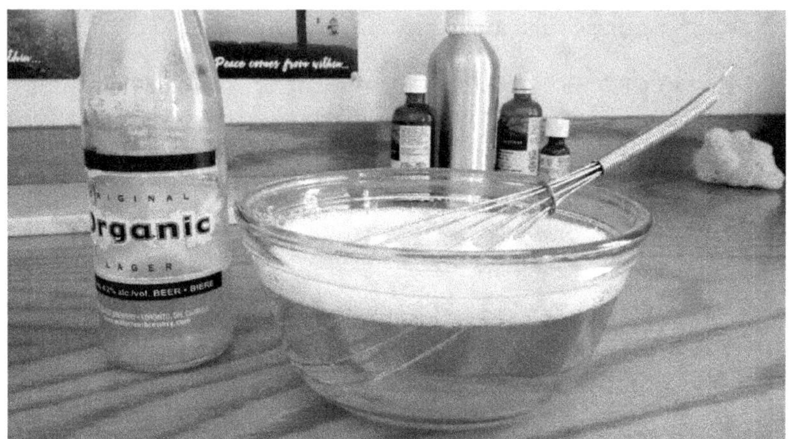

Including beer in your homemade shampoo helps to promote the health, color and growth rate of your hair. It is even helpful in controlling dandruff. There are very few ingredients needed for this DIY recipe, so it's easy to make, too.

Makes about 1 cup finished

Prep Time: 35 minutes

Ingredients:

- 1 cup of beer, any type
- 1 cup mild shampoo from your supply of homemade shampoos

Instructions:

1. Boil the beer for about 13-15 minutes. It should reduce to about 1/2 cup.

2. Measure a cup of mild shampoo into medium sized bowl.

3. Remove pan from heat and cool for 5-10 minutes.

4. Pour the beer into the bowl with the shampoo.

5. Transfer conditioner to lidded plastic container. Use as needed.

14 – DIY Coconut & Tea Tree Oil Shampoo

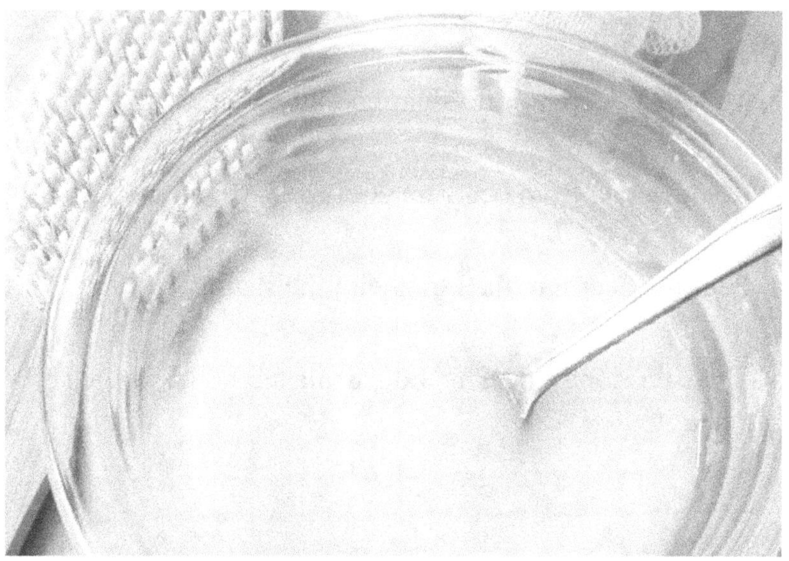

Coconuts are a popular ingredient in natural products made at home. This is actually only semi-DIY, since it includes mild baby shampoo, but it's still a great improvement over the chemicals in commercial shampoos.

Makes about 3/4 cup

Prep Time: 5-10 minutes

Ingredients:

- 1/3 cup of baby shampoo, organic
- 1/4 cup of milk, coconut
- 1 tsp. of almond, vitamin E or olive oil
- 10 - 20 drops tea tree oil

Instructions:

1. Add baby shampoo and coconut milk to plastic bottle.

2. Add 1 tsp. oil. Add 10-20 drops of tea tree oil.

3. Shake to combine the ingredients well.

15 – Homemade Clay Hair Shampoo Mask

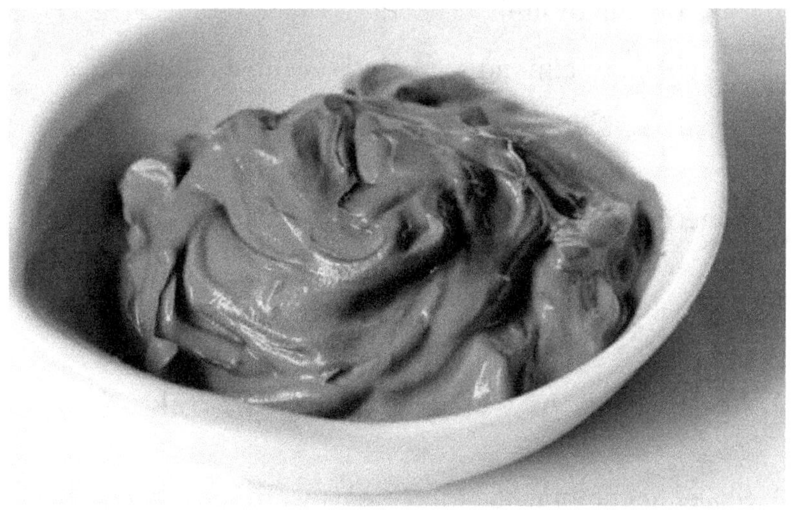

This recipe may even be a bit fun to prepare, and it will leave your hair feeling voluminous and soft when you're done. The mask should be thick, and there must be enough of it to cover the hair completely. After you apply your shampoo mask, leave it on for about 10 minutes. Then simply rinse well using warm water, till the water is running clear.

Makes about 6-8 tbsp.

Prep Time: 35-45 minutes

Ingredients:

- 3-4 tbsp. apple cider vinegar or water
- 3-4 tbsp. bentonite clay

Instructions:

1. Mix 3 to 4 tbsp. of water or vinegar with 3 to 4 tbsp. of bentonite clay. Dampen hair and apply it generously. If your hair is longer, use more.

2. After you apply, leave mask on for about 10 minutes. Rinse well using warm water till water is running clean. Rinse with apple cider vinegar if you like, for extra softness and moisture.

16 – Vegan DIY Shampoo

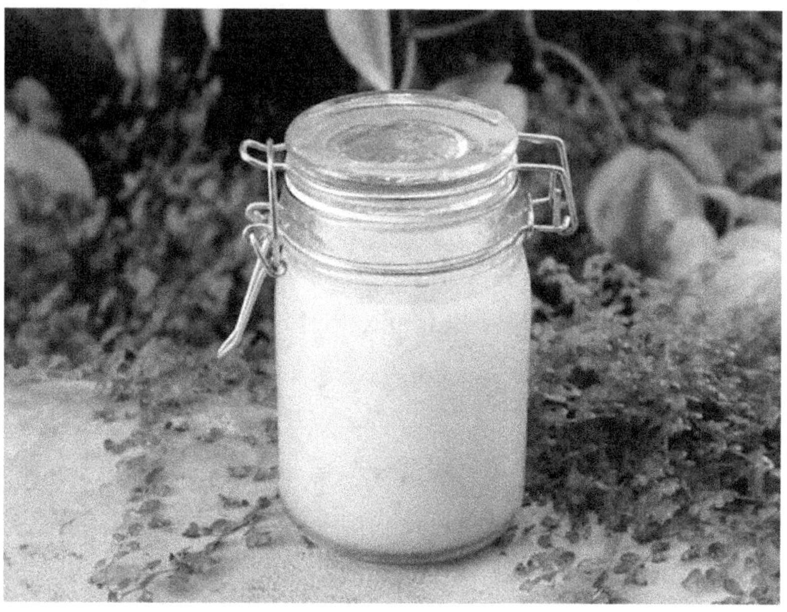

Lots of commercial shampoos add one or even two different types of harmful parabens to their formula. While there isn't a lot of hard science to back up the fact that parabens are harmful, those in the green community and even many scientists feel that parabens can be harmful to the body. There is no need to take that risk. You can make your own paraben-free, vegan shampoo at home, and it's affordable, too.

Makes 2+ cups

Prep Time: 10 minutes

Ingredients:

- 1 cup of water, distilled
- 1 cup of castile soap liquid
- 2 tsp. of grapeseed or jojoba oil
- 1/8 cup of Aloe Vera gel
- Optional: 5 drops essential oil – your favorite(s)

Instructions:

1. Combine all the ingredients. Pour into plastic bottle (an empty, rinsed bottle from your old shampoo is fine).

2. Shake well before using. Apply to scalp. Even though it is thin, it will lather and clean well.

17 – Homemade Ylang Ylang Shampoo

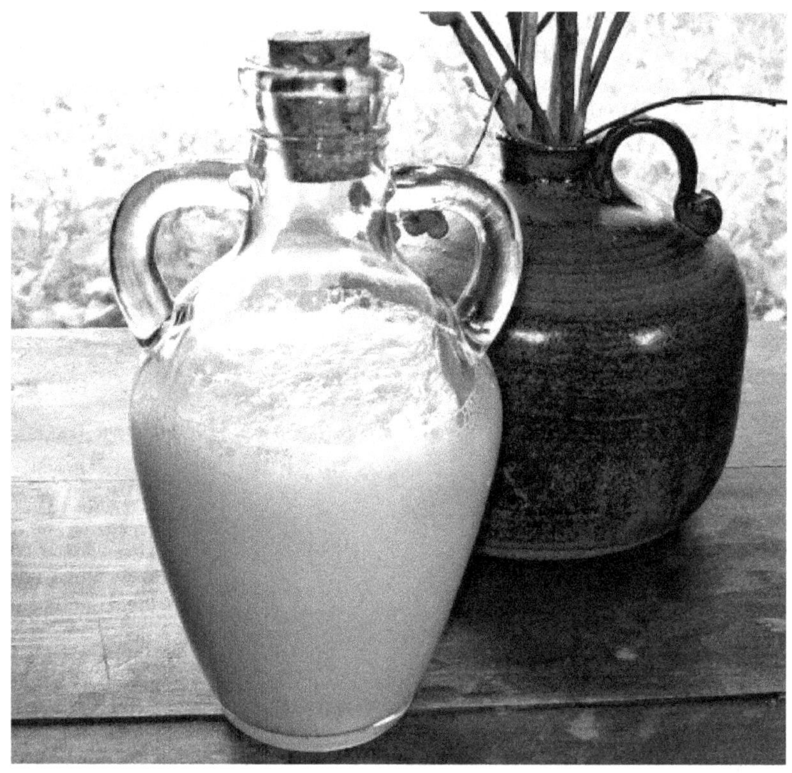

If you have curly hair, your shampoo must keep your hair moisturized properly, without allowing it to build up excessive amounts of oil. This shampoo will help your hair to achieve that balance. It keeps hair healthy and fresh but won't strip it of its natural oils, which are essential to proper health of your hair.

Makes about 1/2 cup

Prep Time: 10 minutes

Ingredients:

- 1/2 cup of water, distilled
- 2 tbsp. of Aloe Vera gel
- 1 tbsp. of almond oil
- 5 - 8 drops Ylang Ylang essential oil

Instructions:

1. Pour 1/2 cup distilled water in a plastic squeeze bottle with a lid.

2. Add Aloe Vera gel & almond oil (jojoba oil is fine, too).

3. Add 5 – 8 drops of Ylang Ylang EO.

4. Mix well.

18 – DIY Chamomile Shampoo

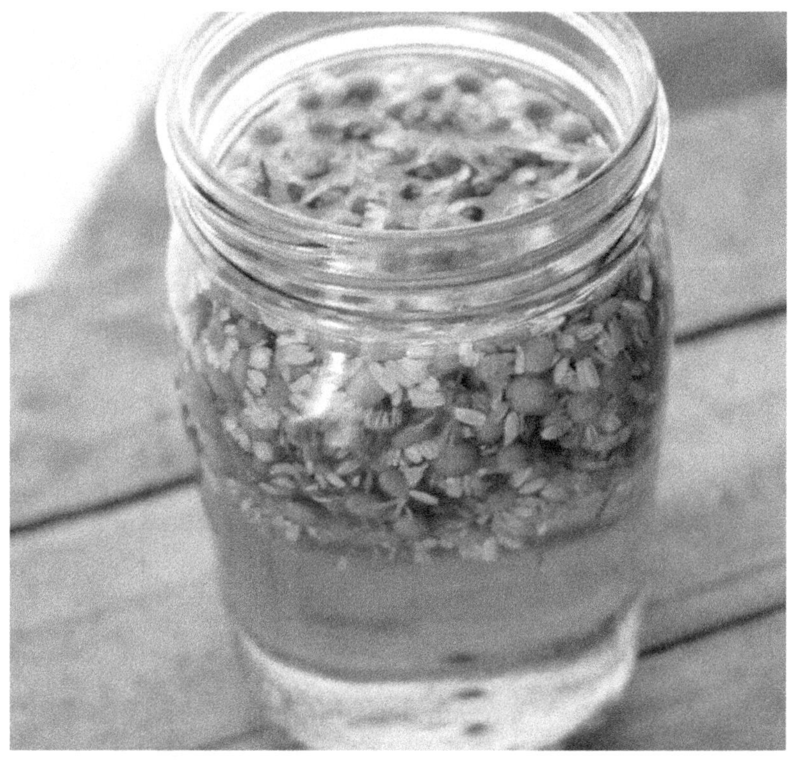

If you use chamomile flowers in this shampoo recipe, you'll note that it turns brownish-yellow. The rest of the shampoo doesn't have any coloring. It won't stain you, and you'll enjoy a thick, nice lather. This shampoo doesn't have a scent that's overpowering, but if you don't like using the flower, you can use less, or use Rosemary.

Makes about 7 ounces

Prep Time: 20 minutes + 3-4 hour setting time

Ingredients:

- 4-5 oz. water, infused w/chamomile herbs
- 2 oz. of castile soap, baby formula, mild and pure
- 1/4 tsp. of oil, carrier (jojoba or almond work well)
- 20-40 drops of essential oil
- A preservative, like Phenonip, Potassium Sorbate, etc.

Instructions:

1. Make herbal infusion: place 1 tsp. of each herb you're using in heat-proof glass or jar.

2. Pour a cup of simmering water over herbs. Cap with saucer. Allow to steep for a few hours.

3. Strain. Set aside four to five ounces. Leftover infusion may be used in bath water. Alternately, you can dilute it with vinegar and use to rinse your hair.

4. Add essential oils, castile soap and carrier oil to water. Stir gently till mixed well. Don't make bubbles if you can help it.

5. Pour into container that's easy to dispense from. An old, rinsed shampoo bottle will work just fine.

19 – Homemade Peppermint & Honey Shampoo

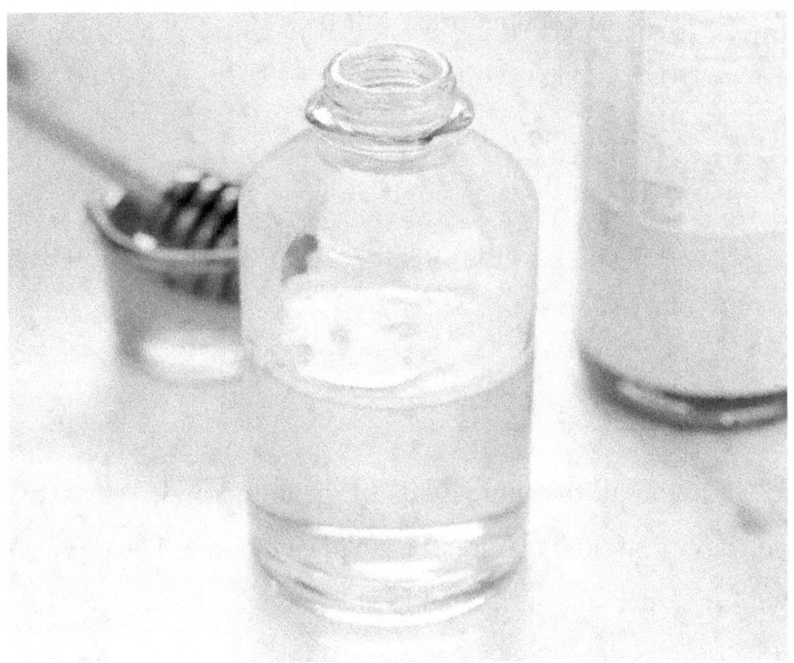

Like many DIY recipes, this shampoo will not lather like conventional shampoos do, but don't let that fool you. It still moisturizes and cleans your hair. Don't apply too much shampoo, or it may leave a residue in your hair.

Makes about 14 ounces

Prep Time: 20 minutes

Ingredients:

- 2 tbsp. of honey, raw, liquid
- 1 can of coconut milk, full fat
- 1 tsp. of castor oil
- 1 tsp. of jojoba oil
- 2 tbsp. of vinegar, apple cider
- 1 tsp. of essential oils - cedarwood, peppermint or clary sage

Instructions:

1. Combine all the ingredients in medium bowl. Whisk till you have a smooth texture. Add to plastic bottle. The mixture will separate, so you'll need to shake it well before you use it.

2. Massage a little shampoo in your scalp. Comb through your hair and leave it on for several minutes. Rinse it off.

20 – Safe DIY Shampoo for Kids

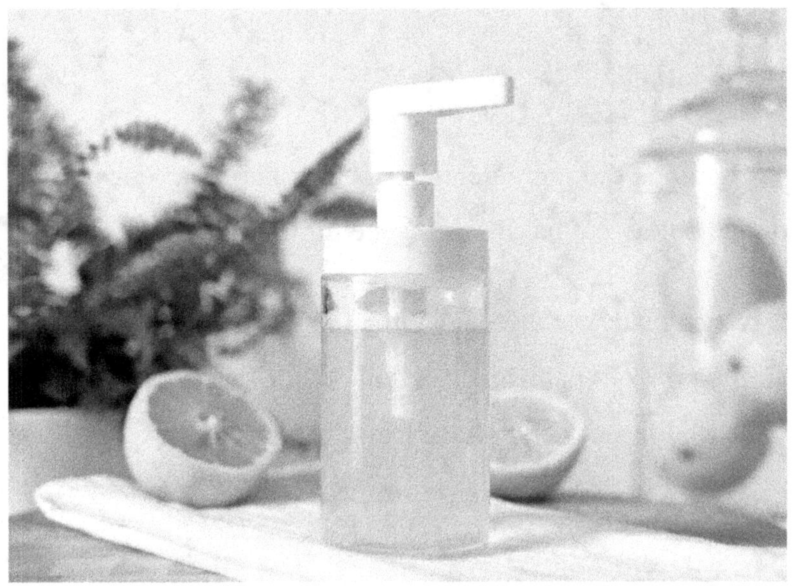

Little heads need a gentle shampoo that won't injure hair, and won't sting little eyes. This is a perfect shampoo for the young ones in your family.

Makes about 3/4 cup

Prep Time: 10 minutes

Ingredients:

- 1/2 cup of water, filtered
- 1/4 cup of castile soap

- 8 drops of lemon essential oil

- 10 drops of melaleuca essential oil

Instructions:

1. Combine the ingredients in measuring cup. Pour into 12 ounce bottle that has a squirt type lid. Store in your shower.

2. When ready for use, shake the mixture well. Pour a small amount in your palm and rub it into your child's scalp. Work your way through their hair. Rinse thoroughly.

21 – Herbal Homemade Shampoo

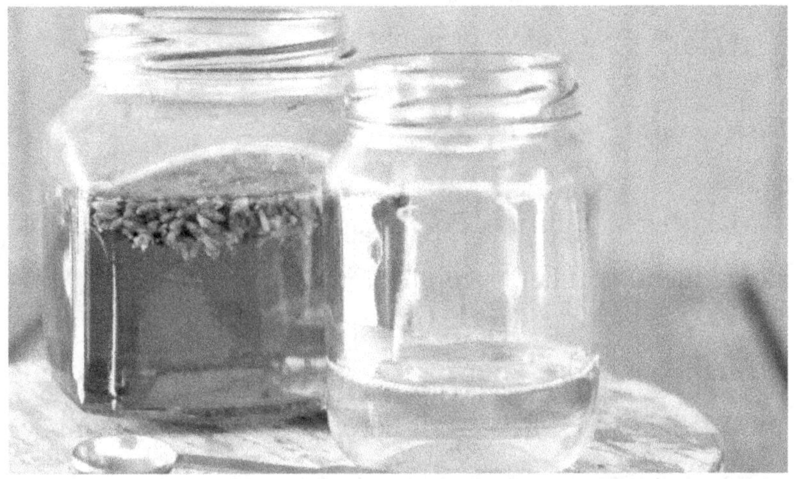

This shampoo is SO much gentler than chemical-laden shampoos. You'll enjoy the scent, too. It's not a shampoo that will leave your hair squeaky, but that's only because it won't strip your hair's natural oils. It still cleans very effectively.

Makes about 11 ounces

Prep Time: 10 minutes

Ingredients:

- 8 ounces of water, filtered
- 3 ounces of castile soap, liquid

- 1-2 tbsp. of your favorite herbs

- 20 to 60 drops of your favorite essential oil

- 1/4 tsp. of olive or jojoba oil

Instructions:

1. Make herbal infusion: Pour steaming hot water over herbs. Cover them. Let them steep for four hours or more.

2. Strain out herbs. Pour reserved liquid in bottle. Add oils and castile soap. Shake well before you use this shampoo, since its contents are prone to separating.

22 - DIY Damaged Hair Shampoo

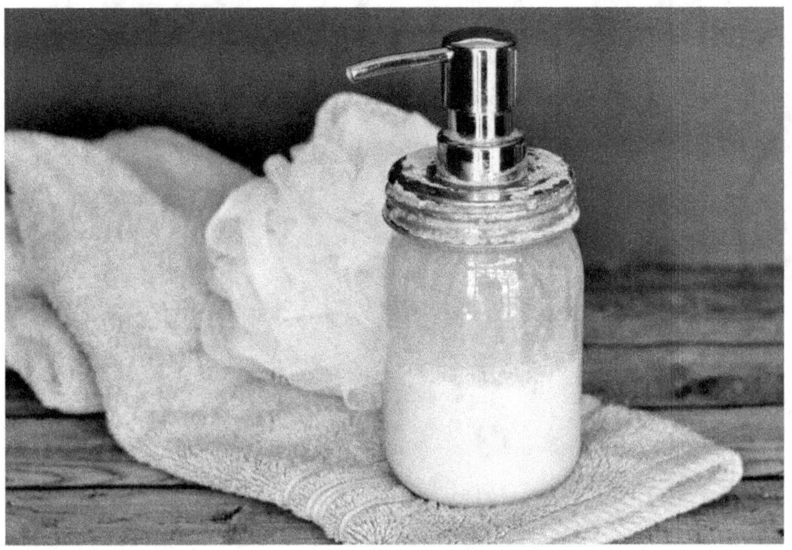

If you've been worried about using harmful chemicals to clean your hair, you may have wanted to "go natural" some time ago. But shampoos that are free from parabens can be expensive, and they may not be able to help conditions like oily hair or dandruff. The answer is making your own shampoos and adding essential oils. This recipe will eliminate harmful chemicals from your everyday showering routine.

Makes about 1 cup

Prep Time: 10 minutes

Ingredients:

- 1/4 cup of canned coconut milk
- 1/2 cup of castile soap, liquid
- 2 tbsp. of coconut oil
- 1/4 cup of honey, pure
- 1 tbsp. of Vit. E oil
- 40-50 drops of essential oils, your favorites

Instructions:

1. Mix the ingredients. Pour them into a plastic bottle.

2. When you begin using this homemade shampoo, be patient. Your scalp needs several weeks to make the adjustment to a natural shampoo.

3. Natural oil will be deposited on your scalp and then your hair will soak up the healthy ingredients.

Conditioners are an important
part of hair care, too. They
help your hair to deal with the
stresses it faces every day.
Here are some of the best DIY
choices...

23 – Avocado Homemade Conditioner

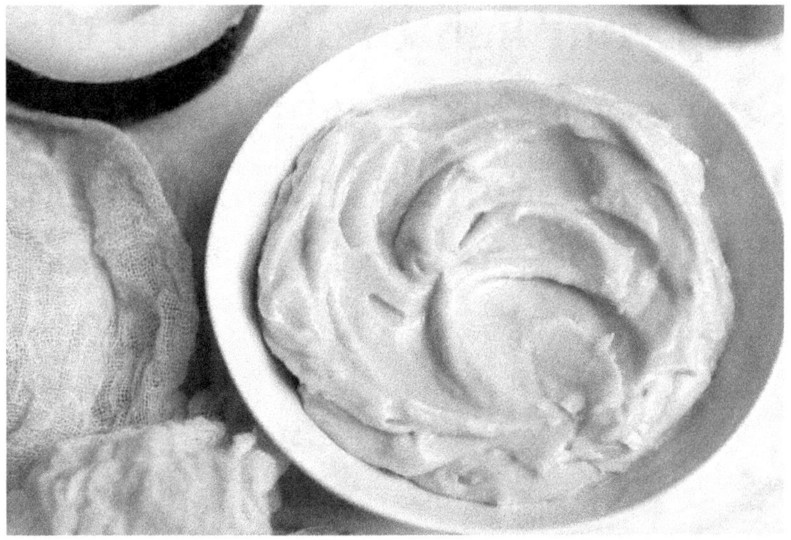

This recipe is easy and quick, and handy for times when you have extra avocados or bananas that you want to use up. Use ripe avocados and bananas, so you can make the most of their nutrients, maximizing the moisture in your hair.

Makes about 5 tbsp.

Prep Time: 5 minutes

Ingredients:

- 1 avocado, ripe
- 1 banana, ripe
- 3 tbsp. of milk, coconut

Instructions:

1. Mash avocado and banana in medium bowl.

2. Add coconut milk. Mix together till combined well.

3. Massage the conditioner into your hair. Leave it on for 13-15 minutes. Hair can be put in towel or clip to help in locking in as much mask as you can.

4. Rinse hair mask from hair. Wash as you normally would.

24 – DIY Herbal Conditioner Rinse

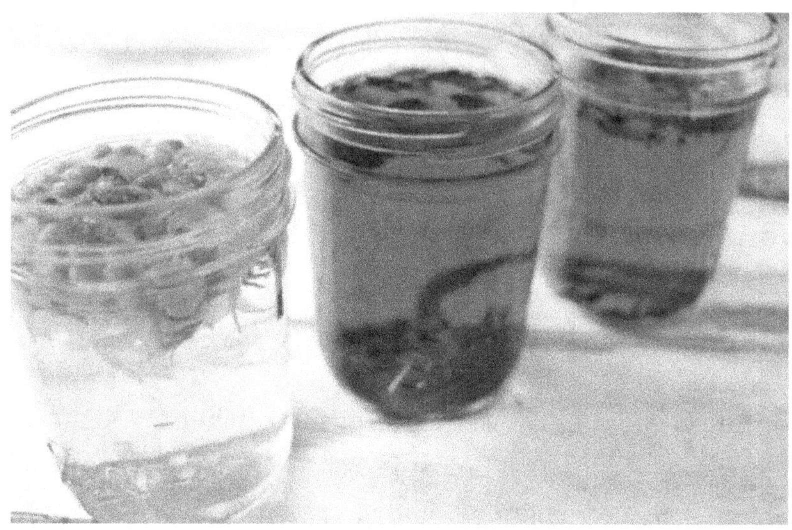

Using an herbal conditioning rinse is among the best ways of using any natural hair care blend available. They are very easy to make, and you'll reap the rewards with softer, shinier hair. When you use a rinse like this after your shampooing, it helps to reduce buildup of product, boosts manageability and balances the pH level in your scalp.

Makes about 1 quart

Prep Time: 40 minutes

Ingredients:

- 1 quart of water, distilled
- 1 large hand-full of lavender, thyme, nettle and rosemary
- 1 tbsp. of lemon juice or apple cider vinegar

Instructions:

1. Bring distilled water to boil. Add herb mixture. Stir, then cover. Allow to steep for 1/2 hour.

2. Strain. Add lemon juice or vinegar. After you shampoo and condition, squeeze the excess water out. Pour liquid on your hair. Do not rinse.

25 – Homemade Lavender Conditioner Paste

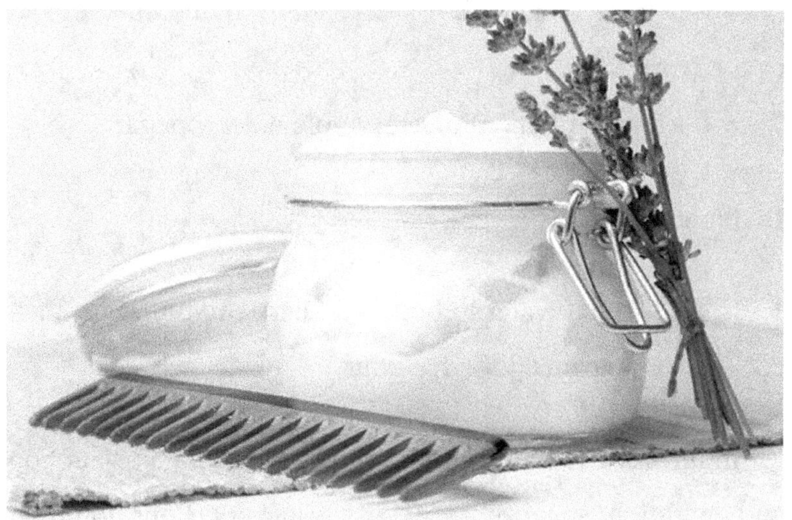

This is a wonderful recipe for moisturizing and conditioning your hair. You can even use it instead of a shampoo, since it cleanses the hair, as well.

Makes about 5 tbsp. paste

Prep Time: 5-10 minutes

Ingredients:

- 2 to 4 tbsp. of water + more if needed
- 2 tbsp. of bicarbonate of soda

- 2 drops of essential oil, lavender

Instructions:

1. Mix all ingredients together. You can add additional water if mixture seems stiff to you.

2. Pour into plastic bottle or jar with lid. Shake mixture well. Apply to your wet hair. Begin at scalp and then work through to ends. Massage in well. Rinse thoroughly.

26 – DIY Hibiscus & Grapefruit Conditioner

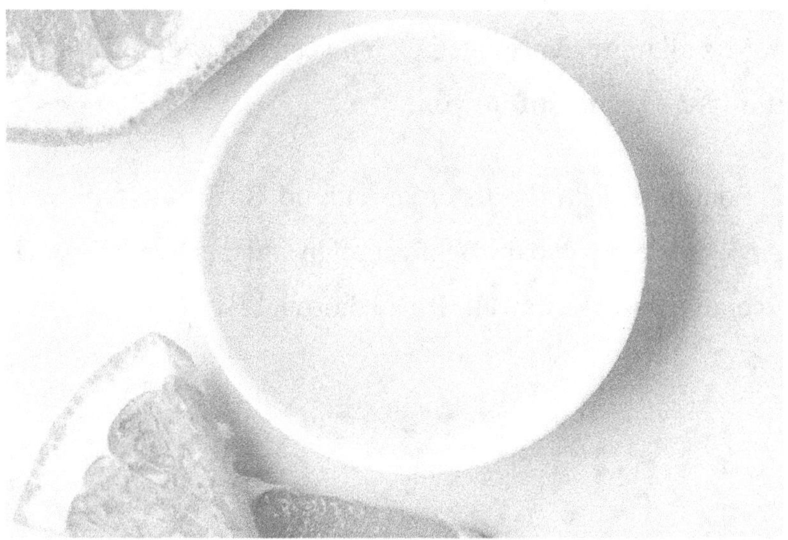

This conditioner is extra moisturizing, so it will help you beat the frizzies. It contains powdered hibiscus, which adds volume and strengthens the roots of your hair. It also **Makes** use of grapefruit seed extract, which is thought to be helpful in preventing damage to your hair from free radicals. Shea butter in an anti-inflammatory, which aids in the treatment of many scalp issues.

Makes about 10 ounces

Prep Time: 10-15 minutes

Ingredients:

- 1 tbsp. of grapefruit seed extract
- 1 tbsp. of powdered hibiscus
- 4 oz. of Shea butter
- 1 tbsp. of essential oil, your favorite
- 2 ounces of Aloe Vera gel
- 3 to 6 ounces of water, distilled or coconut

Instructions:

1. Melt Shea butter in pot.

2. Add remainder of ingredients.

3. Control thickness by adjusting water amount.

4. You can save this batch for up to a month.

27 – Homemade Aloe Vera & Lemon Conditioner

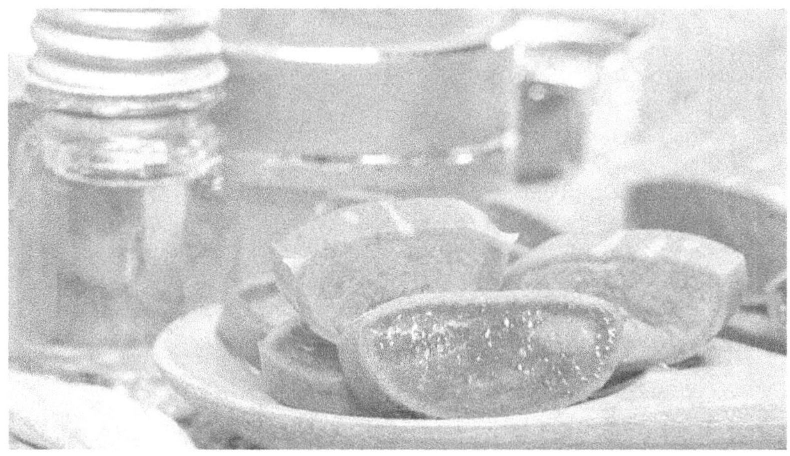

Aloe Vera is able to stimulate the growth of healthy hair, and bring it new shine. It also restores your hair's pH balance.

Makes about 8 tbsp.

Prep Time: 5 minutes

Ingredients:

- 4 tbsp. or more of natural aloe Vera gel
- 4 tbsp. of lemon juice, fresh

Instructions:

1. Combine Aloe Vera and lemon juice in medium sized bowl.

2. Apply to shampooed and rinsed hair. Leave on for about five minutes or so.

3. Rinse with warm water.

28 – DIY Sensitive Scalp Conditioner

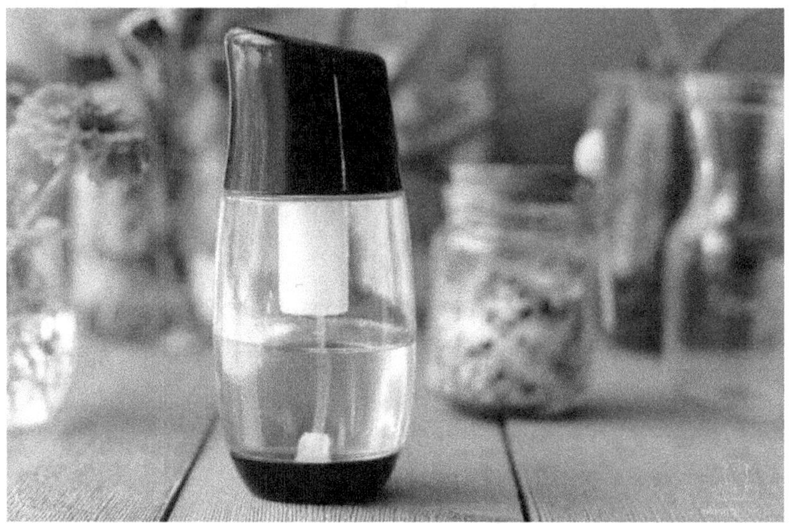

The vegetable glycerin in this conditioner is a natural moisturizer, which leaves your hair softer, all day long. It does best when you combine it with essential oils like rosemary, peppermint or lavender.

Makes about 1/2 cup

Prep Time: 5 minutes

Ingredients:

- 1/2 cup of water, distilled
- 10 drops of essential oil, your favorite

- 10 drops of glycerin, vegetable

Instructions:

1. Pour all ingredients in small bottle.

2. Shake well. Apply to scalp and hair.

3. Leave conditioner in for five minutes or more.

4. You can use this batch for up to two weeks or so.

29 – Homemade Yogurt & Egg Conditioner

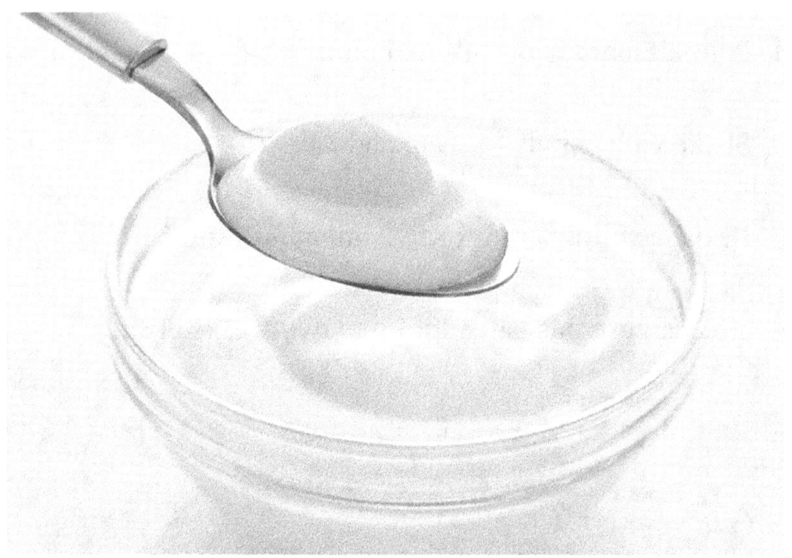

Yogurt is an easy way to help the health of your hair. It has lactic acid and protein, which are especially beneficial in scalp cleansing.

Makes about 10 tbsp.

Prep Time: 5 minutes

Ingredients:

- 6 tbsp. yogurt, plain
- 1 egg, large

Instructions:

1. Beat one large egg into a medium bowl. Add 6 tbsp. yogurt. Mix well.

2. Massage conditioner on hair. Keep covered. Leave in for 15 to 30 minutes. Rinse well.

30 – Damage Control DIY Conditioner

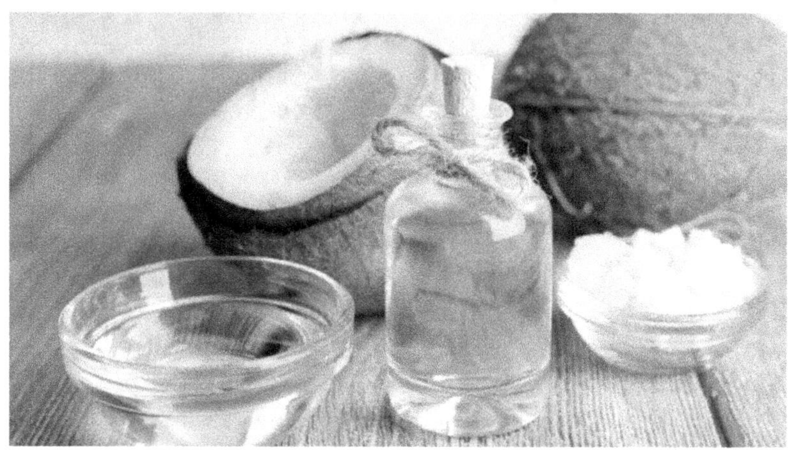

This homemade, natural hair conditioner uses Aloe Vera juice, coconut oil, and any other of your favorite essential oils. These ingredients combine to prevent hair breakage, scalp itch and split ends.

Makes about 14 tbsp.

Prep Time: 10-15 minutes

Ingredients:

- 2 to 4 tbsp. of coconut water
- 2 tbsp. of Aloe Vera juice

- 2 tbsp. of coconut oil

- 2 tbsp. of castor oil

- 2 tbsp. of Ylang-Ylang oil

- 2 tbsp. of honey, pure

- Optional: 6 drops of essential oil, your favorite

Instructions:

1. Melt the coconut oil over low heat till it has melted fully.

2. Add in other ingredients slowly.

3. Turn oven burner off. Allow conditioner to cool.

4. Apply to scalp and hair.

31 – Homemade Vinegar & Honey Conditioner

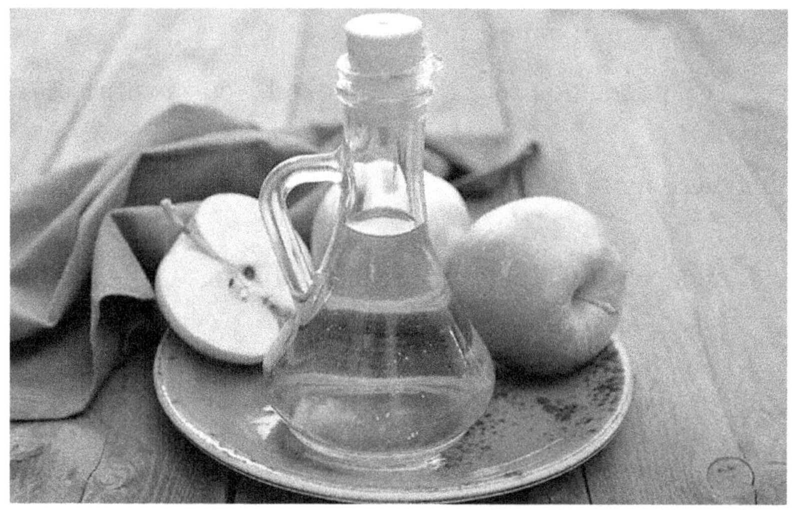

There are numerous positive impacts to using apple cider vinegar as a conditioner. This type of vinegar contains many nutrients that work to build stronger hair, including potassium, B vitamins and vitamin C. Since it's also acidic, it restores your scalp's natural pH. It will make your hair less likely to develop tangles, too.

Makes about 2 cups

Prep Time: 5-10 minutes

Ingredients:

- 2 tbsp. vinegar, apple cider
- 1 tbsp. of honey, pure
- 2 cups water

Instructions:

1. Mix all ingredients well in medium bowl.

2. After your hair has been shampooed, pour this mixture on tips of your hair. It should not be exposed overly to scalp. Don't rinse it out.

32 – DIY Rosemary Oil Conditioner

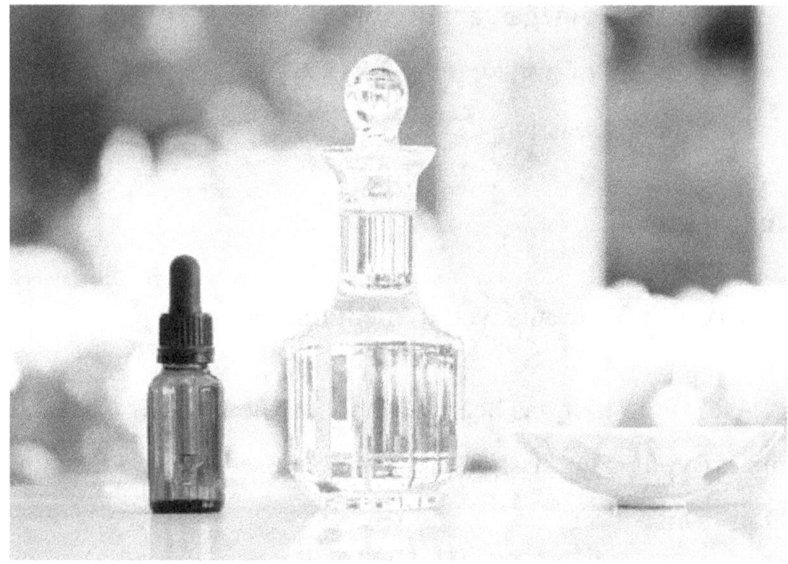

This natural conditioner can be made at home, whenever you have time. It combines sweet almond and jojoba oils, which allows it to promote proper circulation of blood in the scalp. It keeps hair well-moisturized. In addition, rosemary oil helps to stimulate proper hair growth.

Makes about 11 ounces

Prep Time: 5 minutes

Ingredients:

- 1 ounce of glycerin, vegetable
- 5 ounces of almond oil, sweet
- 5 ounces of jojoba oil
- 15 drops of essential oil, rosemary

Instructions:

1. Pour all ingredients into small sized spray bottle.

2. Shake well.

3. Add water till bottle is nearly full.

4. Shake mixture again.

5. This batch will last up to a week or so, depending on how often it is used.

33 – Homemade Honey & Coconut Oil Conditioner

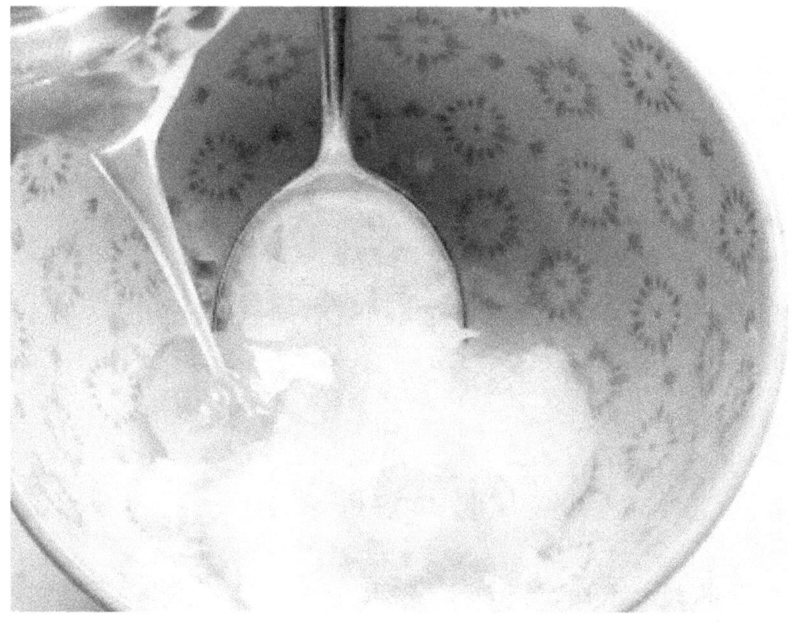

Coconut oil helps hair to become soft and smooth, and it is elemental in helping you to grow thicker, longer hair. The fatty acids and essential minerals found in coconut oil are responsible for nourishing your scalp, too.

Makes about 5 tbsp.

Prep Time: 5 minutes

Ingredients:

- 1 tbsp. of honey, pure
- 1 tbsp. oil, coconut
- 2 tbsp. curd
- 1 tbsp. of lemon juice, fresh
- 1 tsp. rose water

Instructions:

1. Mix all ingredients. Apply on shampooed hair and leave it there for 10 to 15 minutes.

2. Rinse well.

34 – DIY Cocoa Butter & Almond Oil Conditioner

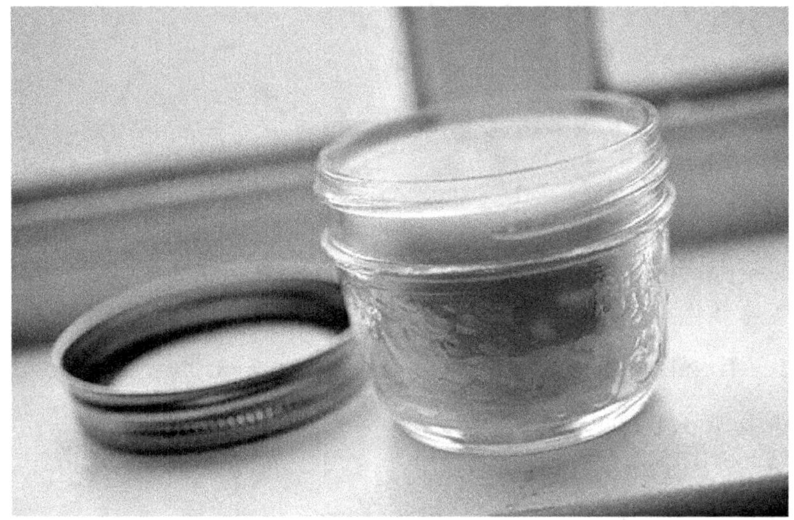

This recipe uses cocoa butter to help soften hair and skin. It's a natural emulsifier, too. The fat content means it can work wonders to revive damaged, dry hair. If you have some left after you condition your hair, it **Makes** a wonderful skin lotion.

Makes about 3 tbsp.

Prep Time: 5 minutes

Ingredients:

- 1 tbsp. of cocoa butter
- 1 tbsp. of almond oil
- 1 tbsp. of coconut oil

Instructions:

1. Melt coconut oil and cocoa butter over pot of steaming water.

2. Add the melted coconut oil and cocoa butter to almond oil.

3. Stir all ingredients together. Pour into small bottle.

4. Apply balm to any damaged ends. Finish with scalp. Leave it on for a few minutes. Rinse thoroughly. You can also leave it on overnight.

35 – Homemade Banana & Honey Hair Mask

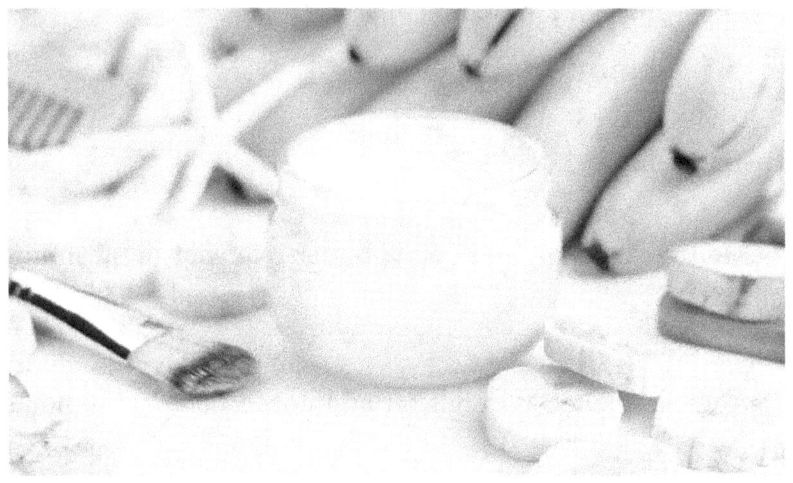

Bananas make excellent conditioner for hair. They are quite beneficial if you have damaged hair, and they work wonders on frizzled and rough hair, too.

Makes about 10 tbsp.

Cooking + Prep Time: 5-10 minutes

Ingredients:

- 1 banana
- 3 tbsp. Honey
- 3 tbsp. milk, whole

- 1 egg
- 3 tbsp. oil, olive

Instructions:

1. Mix all ingredients together well, creating a paste.

2. Apply to hair. Leave in for 20-30 minutes. Rinse well.

36 – DIY Shea Butter Conditioner

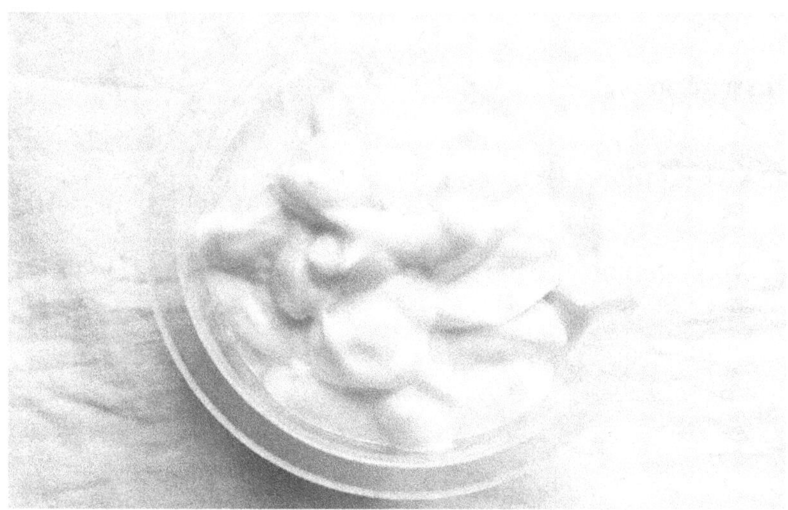

Shea butter is a rich source of oils and fatty acids, both of which reduce split ends and tame frizzy hair. This conditioner keeps hair hydrated well and reduces that drying effect regular shampoos may have on hair.

Makes about 5 tbsp.

Prep Time: 25 – 35 minutes

Ingredients:

- 1 tbsp. of Shea butter
- 2 tbsp. of coconut oil
- 1 tsp. of Argan oil

- Optional: 2 to 3 drops of essential oil, your favorite

Instructions:

1. Warm Shea butter and coconut oil together till you have a fully melted mixture.

2. Add argan oil. Whip all ingredients till combined well.

3. Add a couple drops of your favorite essential oil, if you like.

4. Apply mixture to roots of hair first, then to tips.

5. Once hair is covered fully, allow it to sit for 1/2 hour or so.

6. Rinse well.

37 – Homemade Egg & Vinegar Conditioner

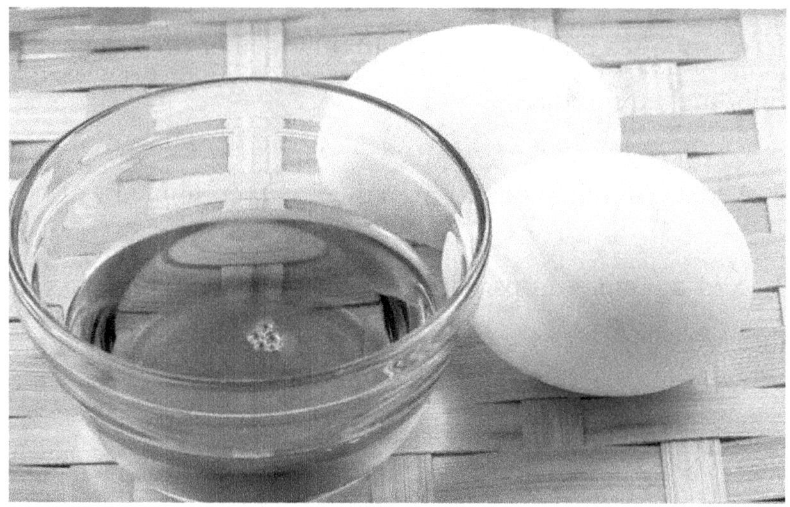

Eggs are effective conditioners and they add shine to dull, lackluster hair. Olive oil **Makes** hair stronger. Honey helps hydrate your hair, while vinegar helps in the treatment of hair loss. This recipe can be used regularly to create stronger, healthier hair.

Makes about 12 tbsp.

Prep Time: 10 minutes

Ingredients:

- 2 or 3 eggs
- 1/2 tsp. olive oil
- 1 tbsp. honey, pure
- 1 tbsp. of vinegar
- 2 tsp. of fresh lemon juice

Instructions:

1. Whisk the eggs, vinegar and lemon juice together. Mix thoroughly.

2. Add 1 tbsp. honey and 1/2 tsp. olive oil. Mix in food processor, creating a thick-textured paste.

3. Apply paste on hair tips. Leave it for 12-15 minutes or so. Rinse well.

38 – DIY Conditioner / Detangler

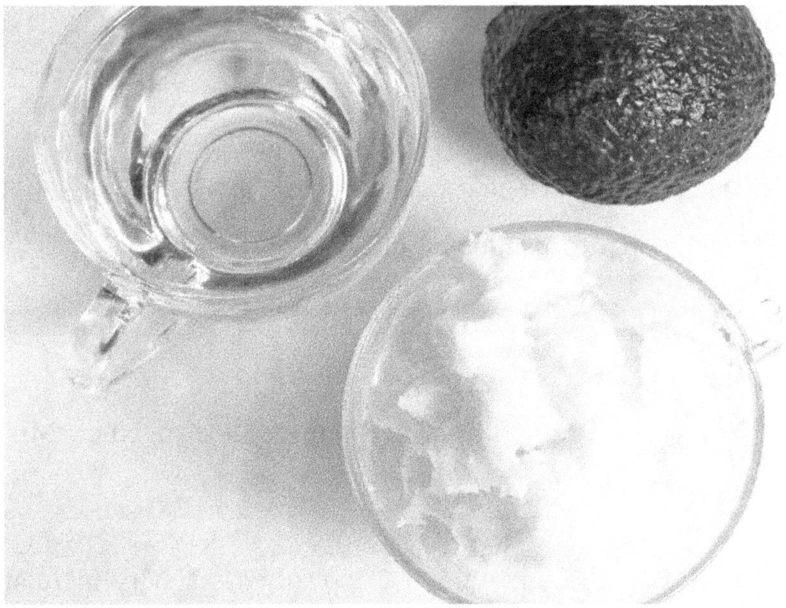

This is a smoothing, wonderful conditioner that will soften your hair and make it easy to untangle after sleep, exercise, etc. It even prevents tangles if you have the problem frequently.

Makes about 25 tbsp.

Prep Time: 40 minutes

Ingredients:

- 8 tbsp. of oil, olive
- 8 tbsp. of Shea butter
- 3 tbsp. of vinegar, apple cider
- 1 avocado, ripe

Instructions:

1. Peel the avocado, then remove the pit and mash it.

2. Mix avocado flesh with Shea butter. As you blend them, add vinegar till the consistency is pasty.

3. Work paste through hair from scalp to ends. Pay special attention to the ends.

4. Put on shower cap and allow paste to sit for 15-20 minutes. Rinse out well with warm water.

5. Leftovers can be refrigerated in sealed container for a week or so.

39 - DIY Lavender Hair Conditioner

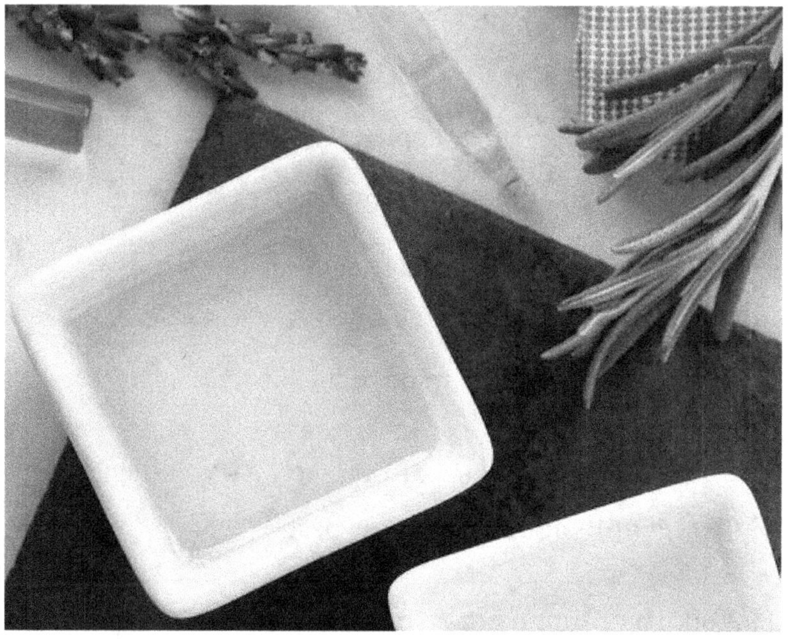

This conditioner will fight dry hair, since it is super moisturizing. It has a wonderful, lavender scent, and the remaining ingredients are helpful for promoting healthy hair.

Makes about 1 cup

Prep Time: 5-10 minutes

Ingredients:

- 1 cup of oil, coconut
- 1 tsp. of jojoba oil
- 1 tsp. of vitamin E oil
- 5 drops of essential oil, lavender

Instructions:

1. Place all the ingredients in bowl of food processor. Mix at high speed for six to nine minutes.

2. Transfer conditioner into plastic container.

3. Coconut oil will melt if left sitting in high temps, so you can store this conditioner in your fridge if you like. You can use it in its liquid form if you don't have to refrigerate it.

40 – Homemade Olive Oil Hair Conditioner

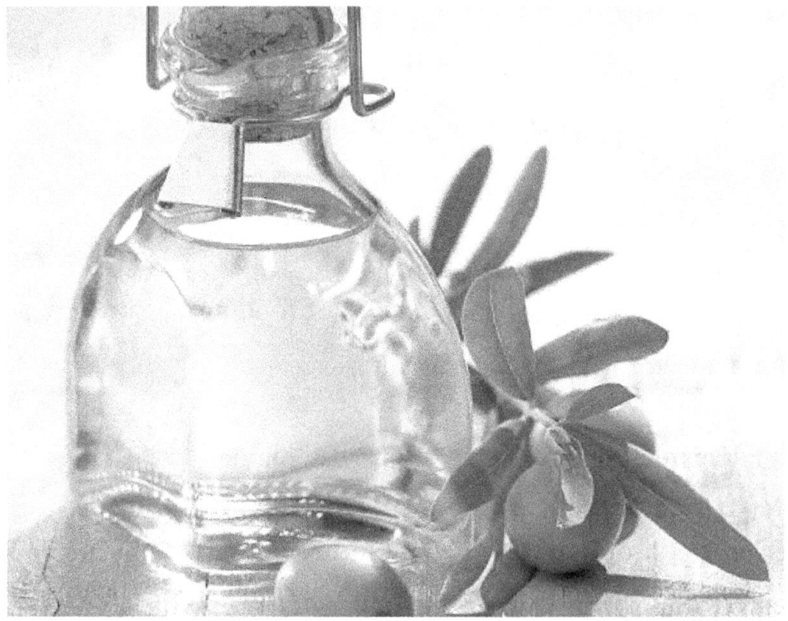

This is one of the most basic conditioners you can find. Once you mix the ingredients, just add your essential oils. It's SO easy to make.

Makes about 4 tsp.

Prep Time: 5 minutes + resting time and warming time

Ingredients:

- 4 tsp. of oil, olive
- 3 drops of essential oil, like vanilla, peppermint, rose, chamomile or lavender, or any essential oils you prefer

Instructions:

1. Drop essential oils into olive oil. Mix gently. Allow to rest for one day.

2. Warm conditioner up a bit before you use it.

41 – DIY Curly Hair Conditioner

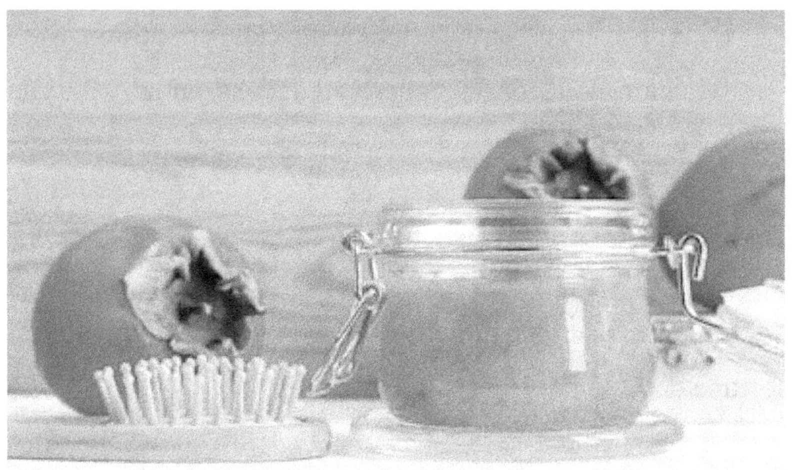

If you tend to have frizzy, curly, dry hair, you will need to pay close attention to its maintenance. This natural recipe will help give you softer hair.

Makes about 1 cup

Prep Time: 15 minutes

Ingredients:

- 1 persimmon, ripe (3/4 cup of pulp)
- 1 Rosemary twig
- 4 tbsp. of oil, almond

- 8 tbsp. of honey, organic

- 8 drops of fragrance oil – some that work well in this recipe include lavender, peppermint, vanilla and chamomile

Instructions:

1. Slice persimmon in pieces. Place in food processor. Mash into pulp.

2. While still blending slowly, add oils, rosemary and honey till the consistency is creamy and mushy.

3. Work pulp through hair. Begin at scalp level. Work slowly through to ends of hair.

4. Allow it to sit for 8-10 minutes in your hair. Rinse using warm water.

Conclusion

This hair care recipe book has shown you…

…How to use different natural ingredients to clean your hair, without the harmful chemicals used in commercial shampoo brands.

How can you include DIY recipes in your hair care regimen?

You can…

- Use apple cider vinegar, which has been used as a conditioner for many years. The scent isn't appealing, but the effects are wonderful.
- Learn to clean and condition hair with essential oils, which are widely used in DIY natural hair care products.
- Enjoy making all kinds of shampoos and conditioners with honey and lemon juice, which make your hair healthier. There are SO many ways to make great DIY hair care products.
- Make shampoos and conditioners using naturally rich ingredients, which are often used in DIY hair care products.

- Make various types of conditioners like masks and other hair care specialties with coconut oil, which is so beneficial to healthy hair.

Have fun experimenting! Enjoy the results!